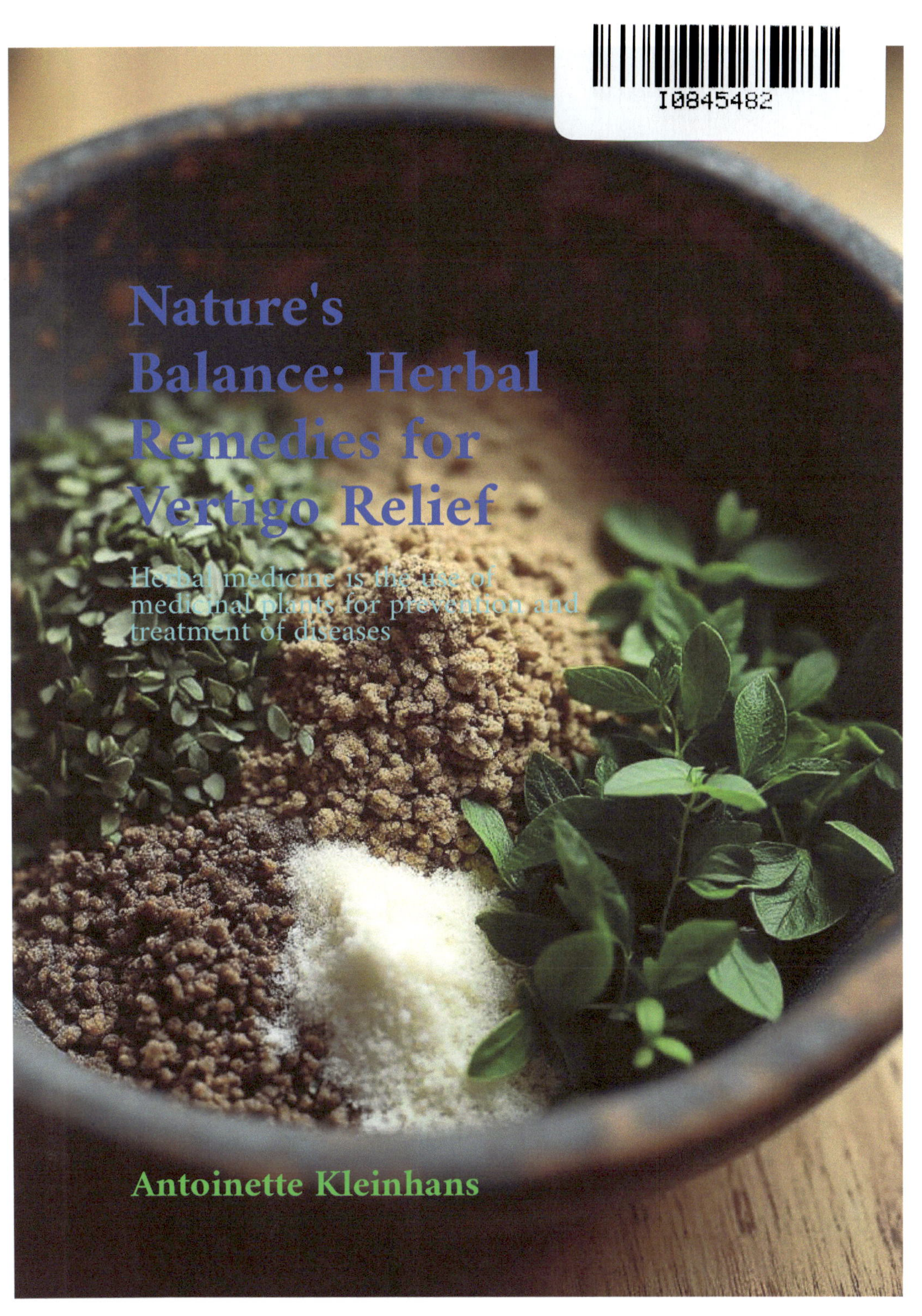

Nature's Balance: Herbal Remedies for Vertigo Relief

Herbal medicine is the use of medicinal plants for prevention and treatment of diseases

Antoinette Kleinhans

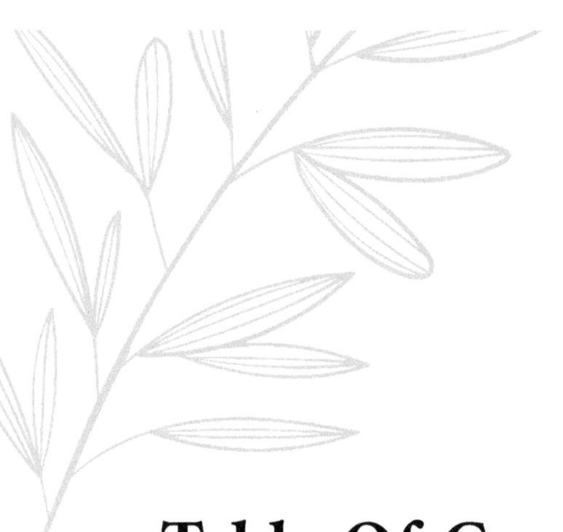

Table Of Contents

Nature's Balance: Herbal Remedies for Vertigo Relief

01

Chapter 1: Understanding Vertigo

The Nature of Vertigo

Vertigo is a complex sensation that can profoundly affect an individual's perception of their surroundings. It is often described as a feeling of spinning or dizziness, making it seem as though the environment is in motion when it is not. This disorienting experience can arise from various underlying causes, including vestibular disorders, inner ear problems, or even migraines. Understanding the nature of vertigo is crucial for identifying effective natural remedies that can provide relief and restore balance to one's life.

The inner ear plays a pivotal role in maintaining our sense of balance. The vestibular system, comprised of tiny structures in the inner ear, detects changes in head position and movement. When this system is disrupted, it can lead to the sensation of vertigo. Factors such as inflammation, infection, or fluid imbalances can interfere with the signals sent to the brain, resulting in dizziness. By exploring herbal remedies that support ear health and overall balance, individuals may find a natural pathway to alleviate their vertiginous symptoms.

Many people seeking relief from vertigo may be hesitant to rely solely on conventional medications, which can sometimes come with side effects. This is where herbal supplements come into play. Nature has provided a wealth of plant-based remedies that have been used for centuries to promote balance and reduce dizziness. Herbs such as ginger, ginkgo biloba, and peppermint have shown promise in addressing symptoms of vertigo. These natural alternatives not only help alleviate discomfort but also support overall well-being.

Incorporating these herbal remedies into daily routines can be an empowering approach to managing vertigo. Ginger, known for its anti-nausea properties, can be consumed as tea or taken in capsule form to help soothe dizziness. Ginkgo biloba is celebrated for its ability to improve circulation, which may enhance blood flow to the inner ear. Meanwhile, peppermint can provide a calming effect and alleviate nausea associated with vertigo. By understanding how these herbs work, individuals can make informed choices that align with their health goals.

Ultimately, the nature of vertigo is a multifaceted issue that can benefit from a holistic approach. By recognizing the connection between the body, mind, and the environment, individuals can explore natural remedies that not only target the symptoms but also promote overall balance. Embracing herbal supplements as part of a comprehensive strategy for managing vertigo can lead to a more harmonious existence, allowing individuals to reclaim their sense of stability and enjoy life to the fullest.

Common Causes of Vertigo

Vertigo is a sensation of spinning or dizziness that can significantly impact daily life. Understanding the common causes of vertigo is essential for identifying effective natural remedies. One prevalent cause is inner ear disorders, including benign paroxysmal positional vertigo (BPPV), which occurs when tiny calcium crystals in the inner ear become dislodged. This misplacement disrupts the normal flow of fluid in the inner ear, leading to false signals sent to the brain about body position. Recognizing BPPV as a primary contributor allows individuals to seek targeted herbal supplements that may aid in alleviating symptoms.

Another common cause of vertigo is vestibular neuritis, an inflammation of the vestibular nerve, often resulting from a viral infection. This condition can lead to severe dizziness and imbalance, making it crucial to explore natural interventions that may support recovery. Herbal remedies such as ginger and ginkgo biloba have been noted for their potential to improve circulation and reduce inflammation, offering a gentle approach to managing the discomfort associated with vestibular neuritis.

Migraines can also trigger vertigo, known as vestibular migraine. Individuals who experience these migraines often report dizziness alongside traditional headache symptoms. The relationship between migraines and vertigo highlights the importance of addressing overall health through natural means. Herbal supplements like feverfew and butterbur are recognized for their ability to help reduce the frequency and severity of migraine attacks, thereby potentially minimizing vertiginous episodes for those affected.

Additionally, anxiety and stress can contribute to feelings of dizziness and disorientation. These psychological factors can lead to a heightened perception of bodily sensations, making it essential to incorporate calming herbal remedies into daily routines. Adaptogens such as ashwagandha and rhodiola rosea may help regulate stress responses, promoting a sense of calm and stability that can mitigate the impact of anxiety-induced vertigo.

Finally, dehydration and poor nutrition can also play a role in the onset of vertigo. A well-balanced diet rich in vitamins and minerals supports overall health, including the health of the inner ear. Herbal infusions, such as nettle or peppermint tea, can not only hydrate but also provide essential nutrients that support bodily functions. By addressing these common causes of vertigo through a holistic approach that emphasizes natural remedies, individuals can find relief and restore balance in their lives.

Symptoms and Diagnosis

Vertigo is often characterized by a sensation of spinning or dizziness, making individuals feel as though they or their surroundings are in motion when they are not. Common symptoms associated with vertigo include lightheadedness, balance difficulties, nausea, and a feeling of disorientation. The experience can range from mild to severe and may be triggered by sudden changes in head position, movement, or even stress. Understanding these symptoms is crucial for both individuals experiencing them and for those seeking to provide support through natural remedies.

In many cases, vertigo can stem from various underlying conditions, such as inner ear disorders, vestibular migraines, or even neurological issues. Therefore, it is essential to identify the specific type of vertigo one is experiencing. Benign Paroxysmal Positional Vertigo (BPPV), for instance, is often triggered by changes in head position, while Meniere's disease may accompany additional symptoms like ringing in the ears or hearing loss. Recognizing these distinctions not only aids in understanding the condition but also guides the selection of appropriate herbal remedies for relief.

Diagnosis typically begins with a thorough medical history and physical examination. Healthcare professionals may conduct specific tests, such as the Dix-Hallpike maneuver, to determine the type of vertigo present. Additionally, imaging studies, like MRI or CT scans, may be utilized to rule out other potential causes. While medical diagnostics are essential, integrating a holistic approach that considers both conventional and herbal treatments can provide comprehensive care for those affected by vertigo.

Herbal remedies can play a significant role in managing symptoms of vertigo. For instance, ginger has been historically recognized for its anti-nausea properties and may help alleviate feelings of dizziness. Other herbs, such as ginkgo biloba, are thought to improve blood circulation, which can be beneficial in cases where poor circulation contributes to vertiginous sensations. Exploring these natural options empowers individuals to take an active role in their health while seeking effective relief from vertigo.

Incorporating herbal supplements into one's wellness routine should be done thoughtfully. It is advisable to consult with a healthcare professional before starting any new treatment, especially if one is already taking medications or has underlying health conditions. Assessing the effectiveness of these remedies often requires patience, as individual responses can vary. By understanding the symptoms and diagnosis of vertigo, individuals can better navigate their choices and find a balanced approach to relief through nature's offerings.

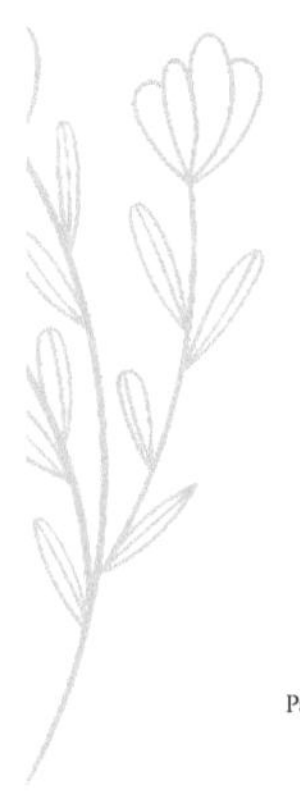

Chapter 2: The Role of Herbal Remedies

History of Herbal Medicine

The history of herbal medicine dates back thousands of years, intertwining with the development of human civilization itself. Early societies relied on the natural world to provide remedies for ailments, with plants serving as the primary source of medicine. Ancient cultures, from the Egyptians to the Chinese and Greeks, documented their knowledge of herbs in texts that have survived through the centuries. These early practitioners observed the effects of various plants on the body and began to compile lists of their uses, forming the foundation for what we now consider herbal medicine.

In ancient China, the practice of using herbal remedies was formalized with the creation of texts like the "Shennong Bencao Jing," which listed hundreds of medicinal plants and their effects. Traditional Chinese Medicine emphasizes balance and harmony in the body, often employing herbs to restore equilibrium. Similarly, the Greeks, with figures such as Hippocrates, advanced herbal medicine through empirical observation and systematic study, establishing principles that are still relevant today. This historical context highlights the long-standing reverence for plants as vital components of health and healing.

As herbal medicine evolved, it began to spread across continents and cultures, adapting to local traditions and environments. In Europe, the Middle Ages saw a resurgence of interest in herbal remedies, often intertwined with folklore and homeopathy. Monastic gardens became centers for cultivating medicinal plants, where monks meticulously documented their healing properties. This period also saw the introduction of herbal texts that compiled knowledge from various cultures, fostering an exchange of ideas that enriched the practice of herbal medicine.

The advent of modern science in the 19th and 20th centuries brought both challenges and opportunities for herbal medicine. While the rise of pharmaceuticals led to a decline in the popularity of herbal remedies, it also prompted a renewed interest in the therapeutic potential of plants. Researchers began to investigate the active compounds within herbs, validating many traditional uses through scientific methods. This shift allowed herbal medicine to regain credibility, leading to a resurgence in its application as a complementary approach to health.

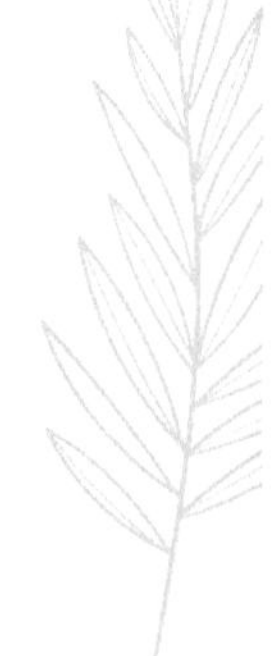

Today, herbal medicine is experiencing a renaissance, with increasing numbers of people seeking natural remedies for various conditions, including vertigo. As evidence of the effectiveness of certain herbs grows, the integration of herbal supplements into modern healthcare continues to gain traction. This historical journey not only illustrates the enduring nature of herbal medicine but also reinforces its significance in contemporary wellness practices, particularly for those exploring natural relief options for conditions like vertigo. The knowledge passed down through generations, combined with modern scientific validation, positions herbal medicine as a valuable resource for achieving balance and health in today's world.

How Herbal Remedies Work

Herbal remedies have been used for centuries across various cultures to promote health and well-being. Understanding how these natural solutions work can help demystify their effectiveness, especially in addressing conditions such as vertigo. The primary mechanisms through which herbal remedies operate include their biochemical interactions in the body, their ability to support bodily systems, and their role in promoting balance and harmony. By tapping into the natural properties of plants, these remedies can provide relief from the disorienting symptoms of vertigo.

Many herbal remedies contain active compounds that interact with the body's physiology. For instance, ginkgo biloba is often cited for its potential to improve blood circulation, which can be beneficial for individuals experiencing vertigo related to inner ear issues or insufficient blood flow. The flavonoids present in ginkgo can enhance microcirculation, thus potentially alleviating symptoms by ensuring that the brain and inner ear receive adequate oxygen and nutrients. Similarly, herbs like ginger have anti-inflammatory properties that can help reduce nausea associated with vertigo, making them effective allies during episodes.

In addition to their direct biochemical effects, herbal remedies also bolster the body's natural defenses and enhance its resilience. Herbs such as peppermint and lemon balm not only calm the nervous system but also help to alleviate stress and anxiety, which can exacerbate feelings of dizziness. By fostering an overall sense of calm, these remedies can create a more stable environment for individuals prone to vertigo. The holistic approach of herbal medicine recognizes the interconnectedness of physical and emotional health, thereby addressing multiple factors that contribute to the experience of vertigo.

Moreover, many herbal remedies are rich in antioxidants and other vital nutrients that support overall health. Turmeric, known for its curcumin content, has strong anti-inflammatory and antioxidant properties that can assist in reducing inflammation in the inner ear and promoting better balance. By integrating such herbs into one's diet, individuals can not only work towards alleviating vertigo symptoms but also enhance their overall well-being. This preventative aspect of herbal remedies encourages a proactive approach to health, focusing on maintaining balance rather than merely treating symptoms.

Ultimately, the effectiveness of herbal remedies lies in their ability to harmonize with the body's natural processes. Each herb brings a unique set of properties that can target specific symptoms or underlying conditions associated with vertigo. By understanding these mechanisms, individuals can make informed choices about incorporating herbal supplements into their wellness routines. Embracing nature's offerings allows for a more holistic approach to health, emphasizing the importance of balance and the body's inherent capacity to heal itself.

Benefits of Using Herbal Supplements

Herbal supplements have gained significant attention in recent years, particularly among those seeking natural remedies for various health issues, including vertigo. One of the primary benefits of using herbal supplements is their ability to provide relief without the side effects commonly associated with pharmaceutical medications. Many individuals struggling with vertigo experience discomfort from both the condition itself and the side effects of conventional treatments. Herbal remedies, such as ginger and ginkgo biloba, offer a gentler alternative that can help alleviate symptoms while supporting overall well-being. Another advantage of herbal supplements is their holistic approach to health. Unlike conventional medications that often target specific symptoms, herbal remedies can work on multiple levels to promote balance in the body. For instance, some herbs not only help reduce dizziness but also enhance circulation and support neurological health. This multifaceted action can be particularly beneficial for those experiencing recurrent episodes of vertigo, as it addresses underlying issues rather than merely masking the symptoms. Herbal supplements are also widely accessible and can be easily incorporated into daily routines. Many people find that they can manage their vertigo symptoms effectively by using herbal teas, tinctures, or capsules. This accessibility empowers individuals to take charge of their health and make informed choices about their treatment options. Furthermore, the growing interest in herbal medicine has led to an increase in quality products available on the market, allowing consumers to select high-quality supplements that suit their specific needs.

Additionally, the use of herbal supplements fosters a deeper connection to nature and traditional healing practices. Many cultures have relied on herbal remedies for centuries, and this connection can provide a sense of comfort and trust in the healing process. By choosing herbal supplements, individuals often find themselves engaging with age-old wisdom that emphasizes natural healing and the body's intrinsic ability to restore balance. This perspective can enhance the overall experience of managing health conditions like vertigo, making the journey more meaningful.

Finally, herbal supplements encourage a proactive approach to health. By opting for natural remedies, individuals can explore lifestyle changes that may contribute to their overall well-being. Incorporating herbs into one's diet can inspire healthier eating habits, stress management techniques, and an increased focus on self-care. This holistic mindset not only aids in the relief of vertigo but also promotes a healthier lifestyle, ultimately leading to improved quality of life. Embracing herbal supplements can therefore be a transformative experience, fostering a harmonious relationship between the body and nature.

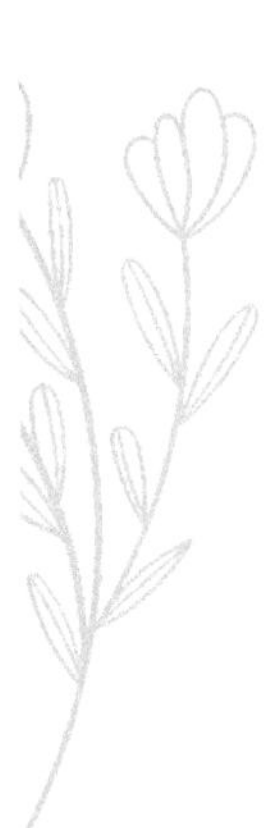

03

Chapter 3: Key Herbs for Vertigo Relief

Ginger

Ginger, a well-known spice with a rich history in traditional medicine, offers promising benefits for those seeking relief from vertigo. This powerful root, scientifically recognized for its anti-inflammatory and antioxidant properties, has been used for centuries across various cultures to alleviate ailments, including dizziness and nausea. The active compounds in ginger, such as gingerol and shogaol, play a crucial role in its therapeutic effects, making it a valuable addition to a holistic approach to vertigo management.

One of the primary mechanisms by which ginger aids in vertigo relief is its ability to improve circulation. Enhanced blood flow can address some of the underlying causes of dizziness, particularly those related to inner ear dysfunction. By promoting better oxygenation and nutrient delivery to the inner ear structures, ginger may help restore balance and reduce the frequency and severity of vertiginous episodes. Incorporating ginger into your daily routine can be as simple as consuming ginger tea or adding fresh ginger to your meals, making it an accessible remedy.

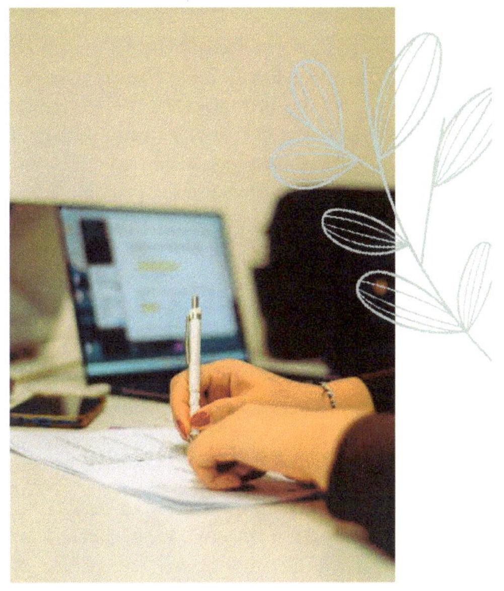

In addition to its circulatory benefits, ginger is also celebrated for its effectiveness in combating nausea, a common companion to vertigo. Many individuals experience queasiness during vertigo episodes, which can exacerbate feelings of imbalance. Ginger has been extensively studied for its anti-nausea properties, particularly in treating motion sickness and post-operative nausea. By alleviating these symptoms, ginger not only provides comfort but also allows individuals to focus on managing their vertigo without the added burden of gastrointestinal discomfort.

For those interested in herbal supplements, ginger is available in various forms, including capsules, powders, and extracts. This versatility allows individuals to choose a method that best suits their lifestyle and preferences. When considering ginger as a supplement, it is important to consult with a healthcare professional, particularly for those on medications or with underlying health conditions. This consultation ensures that ginger can be safely integrated into a broader plan for vertigo relief, maximizing its benefits while minimizing potential interactions.

In conclusion, ginger stands out as a powerful ally in the quest for natural vertigo relief. Its ability to improve circulation and alleviate nausea makes it a multifaceted remedy that can enhance overall well-being. By exploring the incorporation of ginger into your diet or supplement regimen, you can take proactive steps towards achieving balance and harmony in your life. Embracing this ancient herb not only connects you with time-tested traditions but also empowers you to take control of your health in a natural and constructive way.

Ginkgo Biloba

Ginkgo Biloba, a tree species native to China, has gained recognition in the realm of herbal remedies, particularly for its potential benefits in alleviating symptoms of vertigo. Known for its fan-shaped leaves and resilience, Ginkgo Biloba has been used in traditional medicine for centuries. Its therapeutic properties are attributed to compounds called flavonoids and terpenoids, which are believed to enhance blood circulation and support overall brain health. This makes it a valuable option for those seeking natural relief from vertigo.

The mechanism by which Ginkgo Biloba may help with vertigo revolves around its ability to improve cerebral and peripheral blood flow. By dilating blood vessels and reducing blood viscosity, Ginkgo may promote better oxygen and nutrient delivery to the brain and inner ear, areas crucial for maintaining balance. Many individuals experiencing vertigo report a sense of lightheadedness or dizziness stemming from disruptions in these systems. Incorporating Ginkgo Biloba into a daily regimen could potentially provide a gentle yet effective means of reducing these unsettling sensations.

Research has indicated that Ginkgo Biloba may also possess antioxidant properties, helping to combat oxidative stress in the body. Oxidative stress can lead to cellular damage, which may exacerbate conditions that contribute to vertigo. By neutralizing free radicals, Ginkgo not only supports overall health but may also contribute to the stabilization of the inner ear structures. This can enhance the body's ability to maintain equilibrium and reduce the frequency or intensity of vertiginous episodes.

When considering Ginkgo Biloba as a supplement for vertigo relief, it is essential to choose high-quality products from reputable sources. Standardized extracts that contain a specific percentage of active compounds can provide more consistent results. The recommended dosage often varies, so consulting with a healthcare provider familiar with herbal remedies is advisable. This ensures that individuals can safely integrate Ginkgo into their wellness routine, monitoring for any potential interactions with other medications or health conditions.

In conclusion, Ginkgo Biloba stands out as a promising herbal remedy for those seeking natural alternatives to manage vertigo. Its ability to enhance circulation, provide antioxidant support, and promote overall brain health makes it a compelling option. As more individuals turn to nature for solutions, Ginkgo Biloba offers a time-tested approach that aligns with the growing interest in holistic health practices. Whether used alone or as part of a broader strategy for vertigo management, this ancient herb continues to hold relevance in the contemporary quest for balance and well-being.

Peppermint

Peppermint, a popular herb known for its refreshing aroma and flavor, plays a significant role in the realm of natural remedies, particularly for those seeking relief from vertigo. This versatile plant, scientifically known as Mentha piperita, has been employed for centuries in various cultures for its therapeutic properties. Its active compounds, including menthol, have a calming effect on the nervous system, which can be beneficial for individuals experiencing the disorienting symptoms associated with vertigo.

One of the primary ways peppermint aids in vertigo relief is through its ability to enhance blood circulation. Improved blood flow can help ensure that the brain receives adequate oxygen and nutrients, which are vital for maintaining balance and coordination. This is particularly important for individuals suffering from conditions that affect their vestibular system. Incorporating peppermint oil into your daily routine, whether through aromatherapy or topical application, may promote a sense of stability and clarity.

In addition to its circulatory benefits, peppermint is also known for its anti-nausea properties. Many individuals experience nausea as a secondary symptom of vertigo. The soothing aroma of peppermint can help alleviate feelings of queasiness and provide comfort during episodes. Drinking peppermint tea or inhaling the scent of peppermint essential oil can serve as effective strategies to combat nausea, allowing individuals to focus on regaining their balance without the added discomfort of digestive distress.

Moreover, peppermint's anti-inflammatory properties can contribute to overall ear health, an essential factor in preventing and alleviating vertigo symptoms. Inflammation in the inner ear can disrupt balance and coordination, leading to episodes of dizziness. By incorporating peppermint into your health regimen, you may help reduce inflammation and support the health of your auditory system. This could involve using peppermint oil in a diluted form for gentle massages around the ear area or simply enjoying a warm cup of peppermint tea to promote relaxation and healing.

Finally, the use of peppermint in combination with other herbal remedies can enhance its effectiveness in managing vertigo symptoms. Blending peppermint with herbs like ginger, which is also known for its anti-nausea effects, can create a powerful synergy that targets multiple aspects of vertigo relief. By exploring various combinations and methods of consumption, individuals can tailor their herbal approach to find what works best for their unique experiences with vertigo. As you consider incorporating peppermint into your routine, remember to consult with a healthcare professional to ensure a safe and effective strategy for your specific needs.

Lavender

Lavender, with its enchanting aroma and vibrant purple blooms, is more than just a delightful addition to gardens and home décor. It has been used for centuries in various cultures for its therapeutic properties, particularly in the realm of natural remedies. Known scientifically as Lavandula angustifolia, this herb is revered not only for its calming scent but also for its potential benefits in alleviating symptoms associated with vertigo. Incorporating lavender into your wellness routine can provide a holistic approach to managing this often debilitating condition.

The calming properties of lavender are primarily attributed to its essential oil, which can be utilized in several ways to foster relaxation and reduce stress, both of which are crucial in managing vertigo. When experiencing vertigo, anxiety can exacerbate the sensation of dizziness, creating a challenging cycle. Lavender essential oil can be diffused in the air, added to bathwater, or applied topically when diluted with a carrier oil, offering a soothing effect that may help mitigate feelings of unease. The gentle aroma not only promotes a sense of tranquility but can also serve as a grounding presence during dizzy spells.

In addition to its aromatherapeutic benefits, lavender can be consumed as a herbal tea or tincture. Drinking lavender-infused tea provides a warm and comforting experience that may help soothe the mind and body. The natural compounds found in lavender, such as linalool and linalyl acetate, have been studied for their anxiolytic effects, potentially offering relief from the anxiety that often accompanies vertigo episodes. Regular consumption of lavender tea may contribute to an overall sense of well-being, further supporting the body's ability to cope with vertigo.

Furthermore, lavender can enhance sleep quality, which is essential for those dealing with vertigo. Poor sleep can worsen symptoms, leading to a vicious cycle of fatigue and dizziness. Incorporating lavender into your nighttime routine—whether through essential oil in a diffuser or a few drops on your pillow—can promote deeper, more restorative sleep. This practice not only aids in reducing the frequency of vertigo episodes but also helps the body recover and rejuvenate, thus improving overall health.

In conclusion, lavender stands out as a versatile herb with multiple applications for those seeking natural remedies for vertigo relief. Its calming properties, combined with the potential for improved sleep and reduced anxiety, make it an invaluable ally in managing this condition. By integrating lavender into your daily life, whether through aromatherapy, herbal teas, or topical applications, you can create a nurturing environment that supports your body's natural balance and resilience against vertigo. Embracing the healing qualities of lavender may lead to a more centered and harmonious experience, allowing you to navigate the challenges of vertigo with greater ease.

Rosemary

Rosemary, a fragrant herb commonly associated with culinary delights, holds significant potential as a natural remedy for vertigo. This evergreen shrub, native to the Mediterranean region, is not only a staple in kitchens but also a powerful ally in the realm of herbal medicine. Its history dates back centuries, with traditional uses ranging from enhancing memory to alleviating various ailments. For those seeking natural remedies for vertigo, rosemary offers a unique blend of benefits that may help mitigate symptoms and promote overall balance.

The primary constituents of rosemary, including rosmarinic acid and essential oils like camphor and 1,8-cineole, contribute to its therapeutic properties. These compounds have been shown to improve circulation and enhance cognitive function, both of which are crucial for individuals experiencing vertigo. Improved blood flow can alleviate the sensation of dizziness by ensuring that the brain receives adequate oxygen and nutrients. Additionally, the anti-inflammatory properties of rosemary may help reduce inner ear inflammation, a common contributor to vertigo symptoms.

Incorporating rosemary into your daily routine can be both enjoyable and beneficial. Fresh or dried rosemary can be brewed into a soothing tea, providing a calming effect while harnessing the herb's medicinal properties. Alternatively, rosemary essential oil can be used in aromatherapy; inhaling its invigorating scent may help clear the mind and improve focus. A few drops of the oil can also be diluted with a carrier oil and massaged into the temples or neck to relieve tension, which may further diminish feelings of dizziness and disorientation.

For those who prefer herbal supplements, rosemary is available in various forms, including capsules and tinctures. These concentrated preparations can offer a convenient way to incorporate the herb into your wellness regimen. When selecting a supplement, it's important to choose high-quality products from reputable sources to ensure potency and effectiveness. Always consult a healthcare professional before starting any new supplement, particularly if you have pre-existing health conditions or are taking medications. Ultimately, rosemary represents a harmonious blend of culinary pleasure and therapeutic potential. By embracing this versatile herb, individuals seeking natural remedies for vertigo can tap into its restorative qualities. With its rich history and array of beneficial compounds, rosemary not only enriches our meals but also serves as a valuable tool in the pursuit of balance and wellbeing. Integrating rosemary into your lifestyle may provide the relief needed to navigate the challenges of vertigo, fostering a sense of stability and clarity.

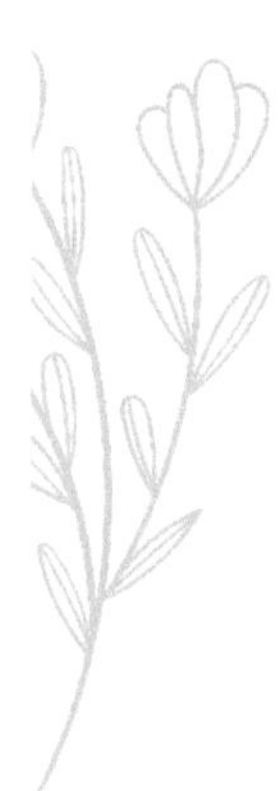

04

Chapter 4: Preparing Herbal Remedies

Tea Infusions

Tea infusions have long been celebrated for their soothing properties and health benefits, making them a valuable addition to any natural remedy toolkit, especially for those seeking relief from vertigo. These herbal concoctions can harness the power of nature to promote balance and wellness. By utilizing various herbs known for their therapeutic effects, individuals can create delightful beverages that not only taste good but also support their overall well-being.

To begin exploring tea infusions, it is essential to select the right herbs. Ginger is a prominent choice, renowned for its anti-inflammatory properties and ability to enhance circulation. When brewed as a tea, ginger can help alleviate nausea often associated with vertigo. Another excellent option is peppermint, which is known for its calming properties and ability to ease gastrointestinal discomfort. Combining these herbs with additional ingredients like lemon or honey can enhance flavor while providing further health benefits, creating a delightful and effective infusion. Preparation of tea infusions is straightforward, making it easy for anyone to incorporate them into their daily routine. Begin by selecting dried or fresh herbs, measuring out the desired quantity, and boiling water to extract their beneficial compounds. Allow the herbs to steep for several minutes, permitting their flavors and properties to infuse into the water. Strain the mixture and enjoy your tea warm or chilled, depending on personal preference. Experimenting with different combinations can lead to unique flavors and enhanced therapeutic effects tailored to individual needs.

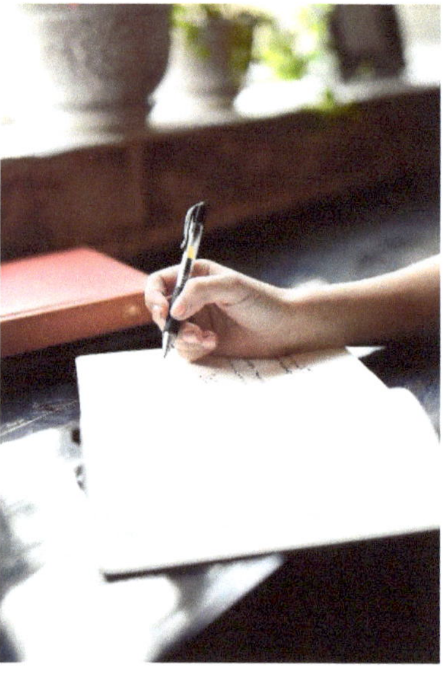

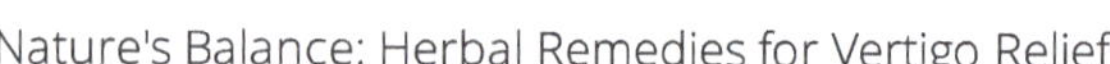

In addition to their immediate benefits, tea infusions can also serve as a form of preventative care. Regularly consuming herbal teas can strengthen the body's resistance to factors that contribute to vertigo, such as stress and dehydration. Herbal teas can also encourage a mindful moment in one's day, promoting relaxation and mental clarity. This holistic approach not only addresses the symptoms of vertigo but also fosters a sense of balance and well-being in everyday life.

Integrating tea infusions into a broader lifestyle that includes proper nutrition, hydration, and stress management can amplify their effectiveness. Consistency is key; establishing a routine of enjoying herbal teas can lead to cumulative benefits over time. As one becomes familiar with their preferred combinations and the specific attributes of each herb, they can create a personalized regimen that aligns with their health goals. Through the simple act of brewing a cup of tea, individuals can tap into the healing potential of nature and find solace in their journey toward vertigo relief.

Tinctures

Tinctures are powerful herbal extracts that harness the benefits of plants in a concentrated form, making them an excellent option for those seeking natural remedies for vertigo. These liquid preparations are created by soaking herbs in alcohol or glycerin, which extracts the active compounds from the plant material. The result is a potent solution that can be easily absorbed by the body, providing quick relief from symptoms associated with vertigo. For individuals looking to incorporate herbal supplements into their wellness routine, tinctures offer a convenient and effective method of delivery.

The process of making tinctures involves a careful selection of herbs known for their therapeutic properties. Common herbs used for vertigo relief include ginger, ginkgo biloba, and peppermint. Ginger is renowned for its ability to alleviate nausea and improve circulation, while ginkgo biloba is often praised for its role in enhancing blood flow to the brain. Peppermint not only soothes digestive issues but also has a calming effect that can be beneficial during vertiginous episodes. By choosing the right combination of these herbs, one can create a tincture that targets specific symptoms of vertigo.

Using tinctures is straightforward, making them accessible for anyone interested in natural remedies. Typically, a few drops of the tincture can be taken directly under the tongue or diluted in water or juice. The alcohol content in traditional tinctures allows for a longer shelf life, ensuring that the herbal benefits remain potent over time. For those who prefer a non-alcoholic option, glycerin-based tinctures are available, providing a sweet and palatable alternative. This versatility in usage makes tinctures an appealing choice for individuals seeking to manage their vertigo symptoms with herbal supplements.

In addition to their ease of use, tinctures can be easily integrated into a holistic approach to health. Combining the use of tinctures with other lifestyle changes, such as dietary adjustments and stress management techniques, can enhance overall well-being. For instance, incorporating foods rich in omega-3 fatty acids and antioxidants can support brain health, while practices like yoga and meditation can help reduce stress levels that may contribute to vertigo episodes. By viewing tinctures as one component of a broader health strategy, individuals can cultivate a more balanced lifestyle.

As interest in herbal remedies continues to grow, tinctures stand out as a practical solution for those seeking relief from vertigo. Their concentrated formulation, ease of use, and compatibility with various health practices make them an ideal choice for anyone looking to embrace natural alternatives. By exploring the world of tinctures and understanding their potential benefits, individuals can take proactive steps towards managing their vertigo symptoms and achieving greater harmony in their overall health.

Essential Oils

Essential oils have gained significant attention in recent years for their therapeutic properties, particularly in the realm of holistic health. These concentrated plant extracts are derived from various parts of plants, including leaves, flowers, stems, and roots. Their unique chemical compositions contribute to a wide range of benefits, making them a valuable addition to natural remedies for vertigo relief. The soothing and restorative properties of essential oils can help alleviate the discomfort associated with vertigo, providing a gentle approach to managing symptoms.

One of the most effective essential oils for vertigo relief is peppermint oil. Known for its refreshing aroma, peppermint has been shown to promote clear breathing and enhance mental clarity. When inhaled or applied topically, it can stimulate circulation, which may help reduce feelings of dizziness and lightheadedness. Additionally, the menthol component in peppermint oil has a calming effect on the nervous system, which can be particularly beneficial for those experiencing anxiety related to vertigo. Combining peppermint oil with a carrier oil for massage can enhance its effectiveness and promote relaxation.

Another essential oil that deserves attention is lavender oil. Renowned for its calming properties, lavender oil can help ease tension and stress, which are often triggers for vertigo episodes. Its soothing scent can create a tranquil environment, promoting deeper relaxation and better sleep quality. Incorporating lavender oil into a bedtime routine, whether through diffusing or adding a few drops to a warm bath, can help mitigate the anxiety that sometimes accompanies vertigo, thus contributing to overall well-being.

Ginger oil is also noteworthy for its potential benefits in managing vertigo. Ginger has long been recognized for its ability to alleviate nausea and improve digestive health, both of which can be helpful in the context of vertigo. The anti-inflammatory properties of ginger oil may help reduce any inflammation in the inner ear, which is often linked to vertigo symptoms. A simple inhalation of ginger oil or its application on the abdomen can provide a sense of relief and stabilize the body's equilibrium.

To fully harness the benefits of essential oils for vertigo relief, it is essential to use them safely and effectively. Always dilute essential oils with a carrier oil before topical application to prevent skin irritation. Additionally, using a diffuser or inhaling the oils directly can enhance their calming effects. As with any natural remedy, it is advisable to consult with a healthcare professional, especially for individuals with pre-existing conditions or those who are pregnant. By integrating essential oils into a holistic approach to managing vertigo, individuals can find a natural pathway to balance and relief.

Herbal Capsules

Herbal capsules have emerged as a popular and convenient method for those seeking natural remedies for vertigo relief. These capsules offer an easy way to consume concentrated herbal extracts without the need for preparation or measuring. By encapsulating the beneficial properties of various herbs, practitioners can harness the power of nature in a form that is both accessible and effective. This method not only simplifies the process of incorporating herbal remedies into daily routines but also ensures consistent dosages, which is crucial for achieving desired results in alleviating vertigo symptoms.

The efficacy of herbal capsules for vertigo relief is rooted in the unique properties of the herbs used. Common ingredients include ginger, ginkgo biloba, and peppermint, each renowned for their ability to support balance and reduce dizziness. Ginger, for instance, has anti-inflammatory properties and may help improve circulation, which can be beneficial for individuals experiencing vertigo. Ginkgo biloba is often praised for its potential to enhance blood flow to the brain, while peppermint is utilized for its calming effects and ability to ease nausea. By selecting the right combination of herbs, individuals can tailor their approach to fit their specific needs.

When considering herbal capsules, it is important to research the quality and sourcing of the products. Not all herbal supplements are created equal, and factors such as purity, potency, and ethical sourcing can significantly impact their effectiveness. Seeking out reputable brands that provide third-party testing and transparent ingredient lists can help ensure that consumers are making informed choices. This diligence not only maximizes the potential benefits of herbal capsules but also aligns with a holistic approach to health, where the wellbeing of the body and the environment are interconnected.

In addition to their effectiveness, herbal capsules can be easily integrated into a balanced lifestyle that promotes overall wellness. For those dealing with vertigo, combining the use of herbal supplements with other natural remedies, such as dietary adjustments, hydration, and stress management techniques, can lead to more comprehensive relief. Engaging in gentle exercises like yoga or tai chi can further enhance balance and stability, complementing the effects of the herbal capsules. This multifaceted approach empowers individuals to take control of their health and fosters a deeper connection to natural healing practices.

Ultimately, herbal capsules represent a bridge between traditional wisdom and modern convenience. They offer a practical solution for individuals seeking to alleviate vertigo symptoms through natural means. By embracing these herbal remedies as part of a broader wellness strategy, individuals can cultivate a sense of empowerment and balance in their lives. With the right knowledge and resources, the journey towards vertigo relief can be both effective and enriching, allowing nature's gifts to play a vital role in enhancing quality of life.

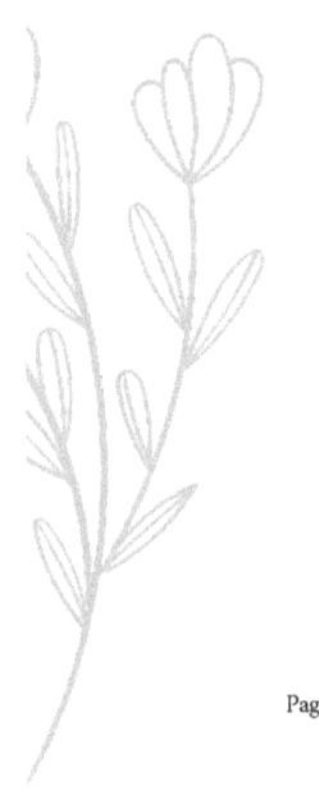

Chapter 5: Incorporating Herbs into Your Routine

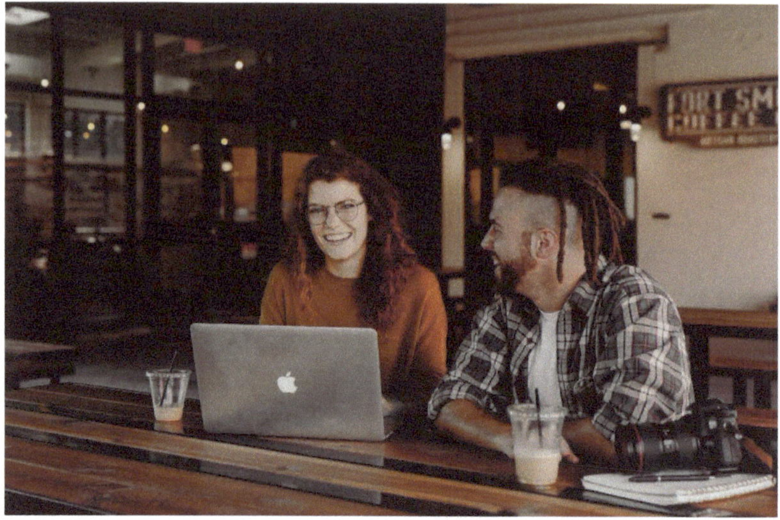

Daily Herbal Regimens

Daily herbal regimens can play a pivotal role in managing vertigo symptoms and enhancing overall well-being. By incorporating specific herbs into your daily routine, you can create a supportive environment for your body to heal and regain balance. This approach not only addresses the immediate discomfort associated with vertigo but also promotes long-term health benefits. Choosing the right herbs and understanding their properties is essential for crafting an effective regimen that aligns with your individual needs.

Ginger, known for its anti-nausea properties, is a popular choice among those seeking relief from vertigo. Incorporating ginger into your diet can be as simple as brewing a cup of ginger tea or adding fresh ginger to smoothies and meals. Its active compounds, like gingerol, help to improve circulation and reduce inflammation, which can alleviate the sensations of dizziness. Consuming ginger daily can also bolster your digestive health, further supporting your body's equilibrium.

Another powerful herb to consider is ginkgo biloba. This ancient herb has been widely researched for its potential benefits in improving blood flow to the brain and reducing symptoms of dizziness. Taking ginkgo biloba as a supplement or in tea form can provide a daily dose of its beneficial properties. Regular use may help enhance cognitive function and balance, making it a valuable addition to your herbal regimen. As with any herbal supplement, it is wise to consult with a healthcare provider to determine the appropriate dosage for your needs.

Peppermint is another herb that can be seamlessly integrated into your daily routine. Its soothing aroma and flavor can provide immediate relief from nausea, making it an excellent choice for those experiencing vertigo. Peppermint tea or essential oil can be used in various ways, such as inhalation or topical application, to help alleviate symptoms. Additionally, peppermint's anti-inflammatory properties can contribute to overall digestive health, which is crucial for maintaining balance.

Creating a daily herbal regimen is about consistency and personalization. It is essential to listen to your body and adjust your intake based on your experiences. Keeping a journal of your symptoms and the effects of the herbs can help you identify what works best for you. With time and commitment, these daily herbal practices can empower you to manage vertigo more effectively, allowing you to embrace life with renewed vitality and confidence.

Recipes for Herbal Remedies

Herbal remedies have gained recognition for their potential in alleviating the symptoms of vertigo, a condition often characterized by a spinning sensation and imbalance. In this subchapter, we will explore various recipes that utilize natural ingredients known for their therapeutic properties. These remedies are designed to be simple to prepare and effective in providing relief from vertigo symptoms, allowing individuals to harness the power of nature in their wellness journey.

One popular remedy involves the use of ginger, which is renowned for its anti-nausea properties. To create a soothing ginger tea, start by peeling and slicing a one-inch piece of fresh ginger root. Boil it in two cups of water for about 10 minutes. Strain the tea and add a teaspoon of honey for sweetness if desired. Consuming this tea twice daily can help reduce feelings of dizziness and nausea often associated with vertigo. Additionally, ginger can be taken in capsule form or used in cooking, making it versatile for various preferences.

Another effective herbal remedy is the use of peppermint, known for its calming effects on the digestive system. To prepare a refreshing peppermint infusion, steep a handful of fresh peppermint leaves in boiling water for 5 to 7 minutes. Strain the leaves and enjoy the tea warm or chilled. This infusion not only helps ease nausea but also promotes relaxation, making it a great choice for those experiencing stress-related vertigo. For added benefits, consider combining peppermint with lemon balm, another herb known for its soothing properties.

For individuals seeking a more concentrated form of herbal remedy, an herbal tincture may be an excellent option. A simple recipe involves using equal parts of dried ginkgo biloba leaves and alcohol, such as vodka. Combine the ingredients in a glass jar and let it steep in a cool, dark place for two weeks, shaking it daily. After the steeping period, strain the mixture through a fine cloth and store it in a dark bottle. Taking a few drops of this tincture daily may enhance circulation and support brain function, which can be beneficial for managing vertigo symptoms.

Lastly, a combination of herbs can be particularly effective. A blend of rosemary, lavender, and chamomile can create a calming herbal bath. To prepare, add a cup of each dried herb to a muslin bag and steep it in warm bathwater. Soaking for 20 minutes can help alleviate stress and promote relaxation, addressing one of the potential triggers of vertigo. The aromatic properties of these herbs not only enhance the bathing experience but also provide therapeutic benefits that support overall well-being.

Incorporating these herbal remedies into your daily routine can empower you to take charge of your health and find relief from vertigo symptoms naturally. Whether through teas, tinctures, or soothing baths, these recipes highlight the potential of herbs to create a balanced approach to wellness. As you experiment with these remedies, remember to listen to your body and consult with a healthcare professional if you have any concerns regarding your vertigo or herbal supplementation.

Safety and Dosage Guidelines

When considering herbal remedies for vertigo relief, it is essential to prioritize safety and adhere to dosage guidelines to ensure effective and responsible use. Each individual may respond differently to herbal supplements, and understanding these variations is crucial for achieving the desired outcomes without adverse effects. It is recommended that users begin with the lowest effective dose and gradually increase as needed, always monitoring for any changes in symptoms or reactions.

Thoroughly researching each herb's properties can help avoid potential interactions with other medications or existing health conditions. For instance, some herbs might enhance the effects of blood thinners or sedatives, leading to unintended side effects. Consulting with a healthcare professional familiar with herbal medicine can provide personalized guidance, especially for individuals who are pregnant, nursing, or managing chronic illnesses. This collaborative approach ensures that safety remains a priority while exploring natural remedies.

Specific herbs known for their potential benefits in alleviating vertigo include ginger, ginkgo biloba, and peppermint. Ginger, often used in various forms such as tea or capsules, can help improve circulation and reduce nausea associated with vertigo. Ginkgo biloba is celebrated for its ability to enhance blood flow to the brain, which may alleviate symptoms of dizziness. Meanwhile, peppermint can offer a soothing effect and may help relieve tension that contributes to vertigo. It is advisable to adhere to suggested dosages, typically outlined on product labels or by herbalists, as exceeding these can lead to adverse reactions.

Another significant factor to consider is the preparation method of herbal remedies. Different forms, such as teas, tinctures, or capsules, can have varying potency levels. For instance, herbal teas may require several cups a day to achieve therapeutic effects, while tinctures may be more concentrated and require only a few drops. Understanding these distinctions can help users make informed choices that align with their preferences and lifestyle, ensuring a balanced approach to vertigo relief.

Lastly, keeping a journal to track symptoms, dosages, and any side effects can be invaluable in assessing the effectiveness of herbal remedies. This practice can aid in identifying which herbs work best for the individual and at what dosages. By maintaining an open line of communication with healthcare providers and being attentive to one's own body, individuals can navigate their journey toward natural vertigo relief safely and effectively.

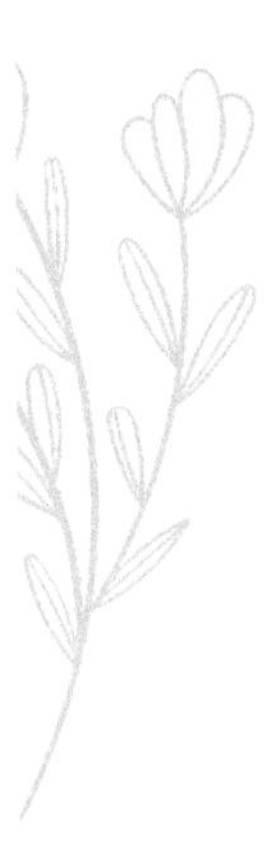

Nature's Balance: Herbal Remedies for Vertigo Relief

06

Chapter 6: Complementary Lifestyle Practices

Diet and Nutrition

Diet and nutrition play a crucial role in maintaining overall health and can significantly impact the management of vertigo. A balanced diet provides the body with the essential nutrients needed to support the inner ear and brain functions, which are vital for maintaining balance. Incorporating a variety of whole foods, including fruits, vegetables, whole grains, lean proteins, and healthy fats, ensures that your body receives the vitamins and minerals necessary to function optimally. Nutrients such as magnesium and potassium are particularly important, as they help regulate fluid balance in the body and support proper nerve function.

Hydration is another key component in the diet for those experiencing vertigo. Dehydration can exacerbate symptoms, making it essential to drink sufficient amounts of water throughout the day. Herbal teas, such as ginger or peppermint, can also be beneficial, as they not only hydrate but may help soothe nausea often associated with vertigo. Reducing the intake of caffeinated and alcoholic beverages is advisable, as these can disrupt the body's fluid balance and potentially trigger dizziness.

In addition to hydration, maintaining stable blood sugar levels is vital for preventing vertigo episodes. Regular meals and snacks that include a balance of carbohydrates, proteins, and fats can help stabilize blood sugar levels, reducing the likelihood of dizziness. Foods rich in complex carbohydrates, such as whole grains and legumes, paired with protein sources like nuts, seeds, and lean meats, can provide sustained energy and prevent the sudden drops in blood sugar that may lead to vertigo.

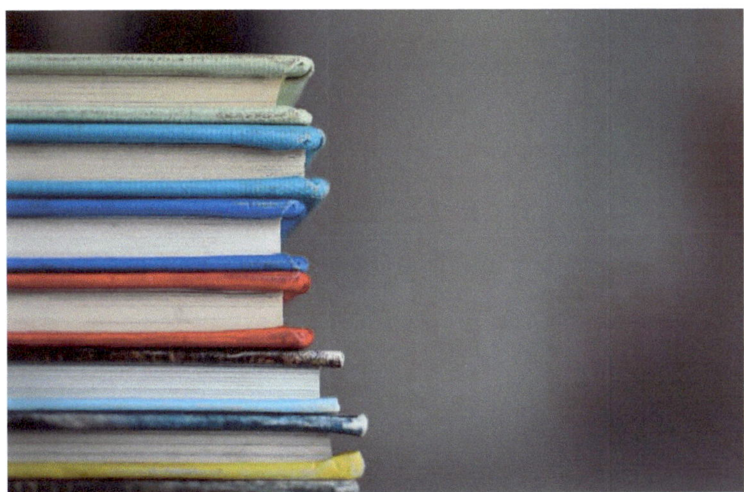

Nature's Balance: Herbal Remedies for Vertigo Relief

Specific dietary choices can also support inner ear health. For instance, incorporating foods high in omega-3 fatty acids, such as fatty fish, walnuts, and flaxseeds, may promote optimal circulation and reduce inflammation. Additionally, foods rich in antioxidants, like berries and leafy greens, can help protect the body from oxidative stress, which has been linked to various forms of dizziness. Including these foods in your diet can create a supportive environment for your body to combat vertigo.

Lastly, it's essential to be mindful of food sensitivities that may trigger vertigo symptoms. Some individuals may find that certain foods, such as those high in salt, sugar, or processed ingredients, can worsen their condition. Keeping a food diary to track your diet and any associated symptoms can be an effective way to identify potential triggers. By focusing on a nutrient-rich diet tailored to your individual needs, you can harness the power of nutrition as a natural remedy for vertigo relief.

Exercise and Physical Activity

Exercise and physical activity play a crucial role in managing vertigo, offering both immediate and long-term benefits. Engaging in regular physical activity helps improve balance, coordination, and overall physical fitness, which can significantly reduce the frequency and intensity of vertigo episodes. Simple exercises that focus on balance and stability can empower individuals to take control of their symptoms, fostering a sense of confidence in their physical capabilities. Incorporating movement into daily routines not only addresses physical health but also promotes mental well-being, which is essential for those dealing with the stress that often accompanies vertigo.

One effective approach is to engage in vestibular rehabilitation exercises, specifically designed to help individuals retrain their balance system. These exercises typically include head movements, balance training, and activities that challenge the body's ability to maintain equilibrium. By gradually increasing the difficulty of these exercises, individuals can enhance their proprioception and reduce the likelihood of dizziness. Integrating these movements into a regular exercise routine not only strengthens the body but also provides a structured way to confront and manage vertigo symptoms.

In addition to targeted exercises, aerobic activities such as walking, swimming, or cycling can also be beneficial. These activities promote cardiovascular health, which is vital for maintaining optimal blood flow and oxygen delivery to the brain. Improved circulation can alleviate some symptoms of vertigo while boosting overall energy levels. When engaging in aerobic exercise, it is important to remain mindful of how the body responds and to choose activities that feel comfortable and enjoyable. This approach encourages consistency and helps to establish a sustainable exercise habit.

Yoga and tai chi are other excellent forms of physical activity for those experiencing vertigo. Both practices emphasize slow, controlled movements and deep breathing, which can enhance body awareness and promote relaxation. These techniques not only improve balance and flexibility but also help reduce anxiety, a common trigger for vertigo episodes. By incorporating mindful movement into daily life, individuals can cultivate a deeper connection with their bodies, making it easier to recognize and respond to the onset of dizziness.

Lastly, the integration of herbal remedies alongside exercise can provide a holistic approach to managing vertigo. Certain herbs, such as ginger and ginkgo biloba, have been shown to support balance and may enhance the effectiveness of physical activity. Combining these natural remedies with a dedicated exercise regimen creates a synergistic effect, allowing individuals to explore various avenues for relief. By prioritizing exercise and physical activity, individuals can take significant strides toward reclaiming balance in their lives, ultimately leading to a more fulfilling and active lifestyle.

Stress Management Techniques

Stress management is a crucial component in addressing vertigo, as stress can exacerbate symptoms and hinder recovery. It is essential to incorporate various techniques that promote relaxation and mental well-being into your daily routine. Mindfulness practices, such as meditation and deep-breathing exercises, can help center your thoughts and alleviate tension. Setting aside time each day to focus on your breath, allowing your mind to quiet, can create a sense of calm that counters the effects of stress on your body.

Physical activity is another effective way to manage stress and improve overall health. Engaging in regular exercise, whether it's walking, yoga, or dancing, can release endorphins and elevate mood. Additionally, activities like tai chi and qigong combine gentle movement with mindfulness, making them particularly beneficial for those experiencing vertigo. These practices not only foster relaxation but also enhance balance and coordination, which can be beneficial for individuals prone to dizziness.

Incorporating herbal supplements into your stress management regimen can further support your journey toward relief. Herbs such as ashwagandha, chamomile, and valerian root have been traditionally recognized for their calming properties. These natural remedies can help soothe the nervous system and promote restful sleep, thereby reducing overall stress levels. It's important to consult with a healthcare professional before introducing any new supplements to ensure they align with your health needs and existing treatments.

Creating a supportive environment can also play a significant role in stress management. Surround yourself with calming influences, such as soothing music, nature sounds, or a peaceful living space adorned with plants. Engaging with nature has been shown to reduce stress and improve mood, so consider spending time in green spaces or incorporating nature into your home. Simple changes, like using essential oils or practicing aromatherapy, can also create a relaxing atmosphere that promotes well-being.

Finally, fostering social connections can significantly impact stress levels. Engaging with friends, family, or support groups can provide emotional support and reduce feelings of isolation. Sharing experiences and learning from others who face similar challenges can empower you to manage stress effectively. Whether through face-to-face interactions or online communities, building relationships can create a strong support network that enhances your journey toward vertigo relief.

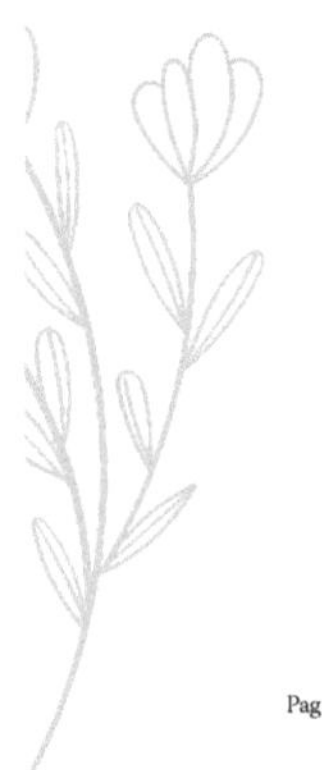

Chapter 7: Case Studies and Testimonials

Personal Stories of Relief

Personal stories of relief can offer inspiring insights into the effectiveness of herbal remedies for vertigo. Many individuals have faced the debilitating effects of this condition, often feeling isolated and overwhelmed by their symptoms. Through their experiences, we see a common thread: a journey toward healing that often involves a deep connection with nature and its gifts. These narratives not only provide hope but also serve as a testament to the power of natural remedies in restoring balance to one's life.

One individual, Sarah, recounts her struggle with vertigo that began after a stressful life event. Traditional medications left her feeling groggy and disconnected. Desperate for a solution, she turned to herbal supplements, particularly ginger and ginkgo biloba, known for their potential to enhance circulation and alleviate dizziness. After incorporating these remedies into her daily routine, Sarah noticed a significant reduction in her symptoms. The ability to reclaim her daily activities and enjoy time with her family without the constant threat of vertigo transformed her life.

Similarly, Tom, an avid hiker, faced the daunting challenge of vertigo that disrupted his passion for the outdoors. Frustrated by conventional treatments, he sought out the wisdom of herbalists in his community. They introduced him to the calming effects of peppermint and the balancing properties of chamomile. By creating herbal teas and tinctures, Tom not only found relief but also rekindled his love for nature. His story highlights how herbal remedies can be integrated into a lifestyle, providing both physical relief and a deeper appreciation for the healing power of the natural world.

Another powerful testimony comes from Mia, who experienced vertigo due to inner ear issues. After extensive research, she began using a blend of rosemary and lavender essential oils, known for their soothing properties. By diffusing these oils in her home and applying them during episodes of dizziness, Mia reported a remarkable improvement in her condition. Her experience underscores the importance of personalizing herbal approaches, as what works for one person may resonate differently with another. It emphasizes the potential of nature to offer tailored solutions that align with individual needs.

Lastly, the story of Alex, a busy professional, illustrates the impact of lifestyle changes alongside herbal remedies. Struggling with stress-induced vertigo, he began practicing mindfulness and incorporating herbal supplements like valerian root into his routine. This combination not only alleviated his symptoms but also fostered a greater sense of calm in his life. Alex's journey serves as a reminder that relief often comes from a holistic approach, integrating natural remedies with self-care practices to create a harmonious balance that nurtures both body and mind.

Expert Opinions

In the realm of natural remedies for vertigo, expert opinions play a crucial role in guiding individuals seeking effective solutions. Herbal remedies have gained traction among both practitioners and patients as viable alternatives to conventional treatments. Many herbalists and naturopaths advocate for the use of specific plants known for their therapeutic properties. These experts emphasize the importance of understanding the underlying causes of vertigo, as this knowledge can significantly influence the choice of herbal supplements. By consulting with professionals who specialize in herbal medicine, individuals can receive tailored advice based on their unique health profiles and symptoms.

One of the most frequently recommended herbs for vertigo relief is ginger. Experts highlight its anti-inflammatory and antioxidant properties, which can help alleviate symptoms associated with motion sickness and inner ear disturbances. Research has shown that ginger can improve blood circulation, which is essential for maintaining balance. Herbalists often suggest incorporating ginger in various forms, such as teas, capsules, or tinctures, to maximize its benefits. Additionally, they recommend using ginger in combination with other herbs, such as ginkgo biloba, to enhance its effectiveness in promoting cognitive function and blood flow to the brain.

Another prominent herb in the discussion of vertigo remedies is ginkgo biloba. Experts point out that ginkgo has been used for centuries in traditional medicine to support cognitive health and enhance circulation. Many studies suggest that ginkgo can help improve symptoms of vertigo by increasing blood flow to the brain and reducing oxidative stress. Herbal practitioners frequently advise starting with a standard extract and gradually adjusting the dosage based on individual responses. The insights shared by these professionals underscore the importance of using high-quality herbal supplements and verifying their purity and potency.

In addition to specific herbs, experts often stress the significance of lifestyle changes in managing vertigo. Nutritionists and herbalists recommend a balanced diet rich in vitamins and minerals that support overall health. For instance, magnesium and vitamin D are essential for maintaining inner ear function and preventing dizziness. Incorporating foods such as leafy greens, nuts, and fish can provide these nutrients naturally. Furthermore, experts advocate for hydration and stress management techniques, such as yoga and meditation, which can complement herbal treatments and improve overall well-being.

Finally, expert opinions emphasize the need for ongoing research and clinical studies to validate the effectiveness of herbal remedies for vertigo. While many individuals report positive outcomes, scientific evidence can further solidify the credibility of these natural treatments. Experts encourage collaboration between herbalists, healthcare providers, and researchers to explore the synergistic effects of various herbs and to develop comprehensive treatment protocols. By fostering a deeper understanding of herbal remedies and their potential in alleviating vertigo, we can empower individuals to take charge of their health through nature's offerings.

Research Findings

Research findings on herbal remedies for vertigo relief have suggested a promising link between specific plant-based compounds and the alleviation of symptoms associated with this condition. Various studies have focused on the efficacy of herbs such as ginger, ginkgo biloba, and peppermint, which have been traditionally used in different cultures for their medicinal properties. These findings offer a foundation for understanding how these natural remedies may contribute to balance and stability in individuals experiencing vertigo.

Ginger has emerged as one of the most studied herbs in relation to vertigo and nausea. Research indicates that gingerols, the active compounds in ginger, can enhance blood circulation and reduce inflammation, both of which are crucial for maintaining balance. A clinical trial involving participants with motion sickness, a condition closely related to vertigo, demonstrated that ginger significantly reduced nausea and dizziness compared to a placebo. Such findings encourage further exploration into ginger's potential as a natural remedy for those suffering from vertigo.

Another herb that has garnered attention is ginkgo biloba. Numerous studies have highlighted its role in improving cognitive function and circulation, which may be beneficial for individuals with vestibular disorders. One study showed that ginkgo biloba extracts could improve symptoms of dizziness and tinnitus in patients. This suggests that ginkgo may help in restoring balance and reducing the severity of vertigo episodes. The mechanism behind this effect is thought to be related to the herb's ability to enhance blood flow to the brain, thereby supporting neurological health.

Peppermint, known for its soothing properties, has also shown promise in alleviating symptoms of vertigo. The menthol in peppermint is believed to have a calming effect on the vestibular system, which could be beneficial for individuals experiencing dizziness. A small pilot study indicated that inhaling peppermint essential oil helped reduce the intensity of vertigo symptoms in some participants. While more extensive research is necessary, these preliminary findings suggest that peppermint could serve as a complementary approach to managing vertigo.

Collectively, these research findings highlight the potential of herbal remedies in providing relief for those affected by vertigo. As interest in natural alternatives continues to grow, it is essential for further studies to explore the effectiveness and safety of these herbs in larger populations. This ongoing research can contribute to a more comprehensive understanding of how herbal supplements can harmonize with conventional treatments, offering individuals a holistic approach to managing their vertigo symptoms.

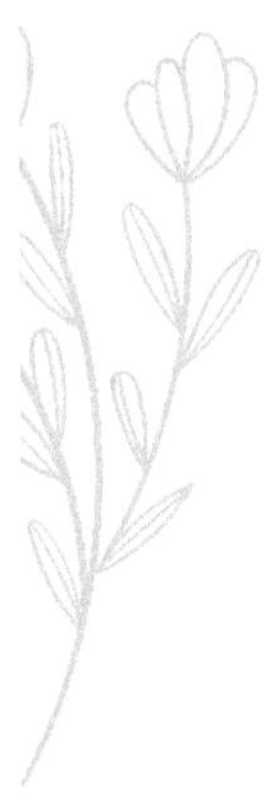

08

Chapter 8: When to Seek Professional Help

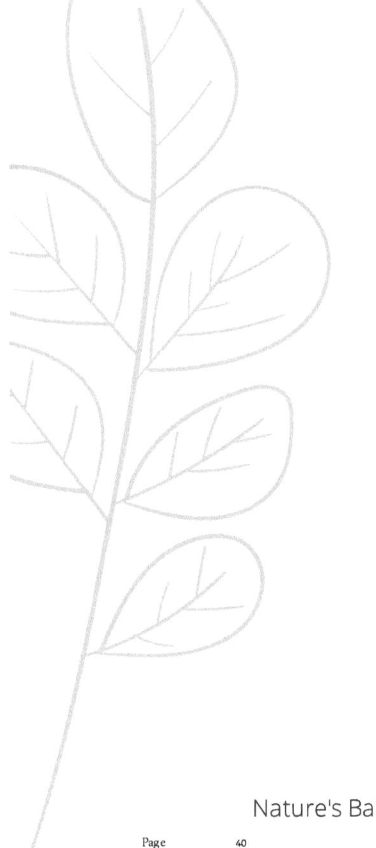

Recognizing Severe Symptoms

Recognizing severe symptoms of vertigo is crucial for individuals seeking natural remedies to manage their condition. While many may experience mild dizziness that comes and goes, severe symptoms can indicate a more serious underlying issue. Understanding the warning signs is essential for determining when to seek medical help and when to rely on herbal remedies for relief. Symptoms such as intense spinning sensations, loss of balance, and debilitating nausea can significantly impact daily life, making it important to pay close attention to these manifestations.

One of the most alarming symptoms of severe vertigo is the sensation of spinning or movement, even when one is perfectly still. This can lead to disorientation, making it challenging to perform routine tasks or even maintain balance. Individuals experiencing this level of vertigo may also find themselves struggling with severe nausea and vomiting, which can further exacerbate feelings of helplessness. Recognizing these symptoms early on can empower individuals to take action, whether that means seeking immediate medical attention or exploring herbal supplements known for their calming effects on the vestibular system.

Additionally, severe vertigo can be accompanied by other troubling signs, such as blurred vision or difficulty focusing. These visual disturbances can heighten anxiety and contribute to a sense of instability. It's vital to note that if these symptoms occur alongside severe headaches, slurred speech, or weakness in the limbs, they may indicate a more serious condition, such as a stroke or neurological disorder. In such cases, prioritizing medical evaluation is critical, and understanding these symptoms can prevent potentially life-threatening situations.

For those who have identified severe symptoms but are looking for ways to manage them naturally, various herbal remedies may offer relief. Herbs such as ginger and ginkgo biloba have been traditionally used for their potential to alleviate dizziness and promote circulation. Incorporating these herbs into one's routine, whether through teas, extracts, or capsules, can provide a gentle approach to symptom management. However, it remains important to monitor the severity of symptoms and adjust treatment methods as necessary. Ultimately, recognizing severe symptoms of vertigo is a vital step in ensuring one's health and well-being. While natural remedies can be beneficial, they should not replace professional medical advice, especially when severe symptoms arise. By being vigilant and informed, individuals can navigate the complexities of vertigo, seeking out herbal support while remaining aware of when to reach out for medical intervention. This balance fosters a proactive approach to health, allowing for both natural healing and safety in the face of challenging symptoms.

Integrating Herbal Remedies with Conventional Treatments

Integrating herbal remedies with conventional treatments can enhance the overall management of vertigo, offering a holistic approach that combines the strengths of both modalities. Many individuals seeking relief from vertigo often look for natural alternatives to complement their prescribed medications. By understanding how to safely combine these treatments, patients can improve their quality of life while minimizing potential side effects. This subchapter explores the principles and practices necessary for achieving this integration effectively.

The first step in combining herbal remedies with conventional treatments is to establish clear communication with healthcare professionals. Patients should openly discuss their interest in using herbal supplements for vertigo relief with their doctors. This dialogue ensures that practitioners are aware of all treatments being utilized, allowing for better monitoring of interactions and adjustments to conventional therapies. It also fosters a collaborative approach to care, where both the patient and the healthcare provider work together to create a comprehensive treatment plan.

When considering herbal remedies, it is essential to choose high-quality products that are well-researched and proven effective for managing vertigo symptoms. Herbs such as ginger, ginkgo biloba, and peppermint have garnered attention for their potential benefits in alleviating dizziness and nausea associated with vertigo. However, the efficacy and safety of these herbs can vary based on preparation and dosage. Therefore, patients should seek guidance from knowledgeable practitioners or herbalists to determine the most appropriate remedies for their specific needs and circumstances.

Monitoring and adjusting dosages is crucial when integrating herbal remedies with conventional treatments. Some herbal supplements may interact with medications, altering their effects or increasing the risk of side effects. Regular follow-ups with healthcare providers can help ensure that any necessary adjustments are made promptly. This ongoing evaluation helps maintain a balance between the benefits of herbal remedies and the effectiveness of conventional treatments, ultimately leading to a more tailored approach for managing vertigo.

Lastly, patients should be encouraged to adopt a holistic lifestyle that supports their overall well-being. In addition to herbal remedies and conventional treatments, practices such as stress management, regular physical activity, and a nutritious diet can contribute to reducing vertigo symptoms. By embracing a comprehensive approach that includes both natural and conventional methods, individuals can empower themselves to take control of their health and enhance their ability to navigate the challenges of vertigo.

Finding a Qualified Practitioner

Finding a qualified practitioner is an essential step in exploring herbal remedies for vertigo relief. As you embark on this journey, it's important to seek out professionals who have a solid understanding of both herbal medicine and the complexities of vertigo. Look for practitioners who hold certifications in herbal medicine or traditional healing practices, as these credentials often indicate a comprehensive education in the field. Additionally, consider their experience and specialties; those who have worked specifically with vertigo patients will likely have a deeper insight into effective remedies and personalized treatment plans.

When searching for a practitioner, you may want to start with local herbalists, naturopaths, or acupuncturists. Many of these professionals integrate herbal supplements into their treatment approaches and can provide you with a tailored experience. Attend local health fairs, workshops, or seminars focused on natural remedies to connect with potential practitioners in your area. Networking within holistic health communities can also yield valuable recommendations, as personal referrals often lead to trusted sources.

It is crucial to conduct interviews or initial consultations with prospective practitioners. During these meetings, ask about their approach to treating vertigo and their experience with herbal remedies. Inquire about the specific herbs they recommend and their rationale behind those choices. A qualified practitioner should be able to explain how the herbs work, potential interactions with any medications you may be taking, and the expected timeline for seeing results. This dialogue is not only informative but also allows you to gauge the practitioner's communication style and willingness to collaborate with you on your health journey.

Before committing to a practitioner, check for reviews or testimonials from former clients. Online platforms and community forums can provide insight into others' experiences and satisfaction levels. Additionally, verify their credentials through professional organizations or licensing boards relevant to herbal medicine. A reputable practitioner should have no problem sharing their qualifications and any ongoing education they pursue to stay current in the field.

Finally, trust your instincts when selecting a practitioner. The therapeutic relationship is pivotal in natural healing, and feeling comfortable and understood can significantly enhance your experience. If you find that a practitioner does not resonate with you or seems dismissive of your concerns, it may be worth exploring other options. Your journey to relief from vertigo should be collaborative, supportive, and empowering, allowing you to reclaim balance in your life through nature's remedies.

09

Chapter 9: Future of Herbal Remedies for Vertigo

Emerging Research

Emerging research in the field of herbal remedies for vertigo reveals promising avenues for understanding how natural substances can alleviate this often debilitating condition. Studies have begun to highlight the intricate relationship between certain herbs and the body's vestibular system, which plays a crucial role in balance and spatial orientation. As scientists delve deeper into the biochemical properties of these herbs, we find a growing body of evidence suggesting that specific compounds may help mitigate the symptoms of vertigo, offering hope to those seeking alternative treatments.

One particularly interesting area of research focuses on ginkgo biloba, a herb long celebrated for its cognitive benefits. Recent studies indicate that ginkgo may improve blood circulation to the brain and inner ear, potentially reducing the frequency and intensity of vertigo episodes. Researchers are now exploring the mechanisms behind these effects, examining how ginkgo's flavonoids and terpenoids interact with the body's systems. This ongoing inquiry not only enhances our understanding of ginkgo's benefits but also supports its inclusion in a comprehensive approach to managing vertigo.

Another area of emerging research involves ginger, a well-known anti-nausea remedy. Preliminary findings suggest that ginger may have a role in treating motion sickness and balance disorders. Some studies indicate that ginger can help stabilize the vestibular system, thus providing relief from vertigo symptoms. As research continues to explore the precise dosages and forms of ginger that are most effective, practitioners are beginning to incorporate this herb into their treatment protocols for patients experiencing vertigo, further solidifying its place in natural remedy discussions.

Additionally, researchers are investigating the synergistic effects of various herbal combinations. The concept of using multiple herbs in conjunction, known as polyherbalism, is gaining traction. For instance, combinations of ginkgo biloba, ginger, and even peppermint have shown potential in preliminary trials. These studies suggest that the combined anti-inflammatory and neuroprotective properties of these herbs might work together to enhance overall efficacy in relieving vertigo symptoms. This approach may lead to more personalized and effective treatment plans for individuals suffering from balance-related disorders.

As the body of research surrounding herbal remedies for vertigo expands, it becomes increasingly clear that these natural solutions warrant serious consideration. The integration of traditional knowledge with modern scientific inquiry holds the potential to revolutionize how we approach vertigo treatment. By continuing to explore and validate the therapeutic properties of herbs, we can empower individuals to reclaim their balance and well-being through natural remedies, paving the way for safer and more holistic health practices in the future.

Trends in Natural Healing

As awareness of holistic health continues to grow, natural healing trends have gained significant traction among those seeking relief from various health issues, including vertigo. Individuals are increasingly turning to herbal remedies not only for their potential effectiveness but also for their minimal side effects compared to conventional medications. This shift reflects a broader movement toward a more integrative approach to health, where each person is seen as a whole, and the focus is on restoring balance through natural means.

One prominent trend in natural healing is the resurgence of traditional herbal medicine. Many individuals are rediscovering ancient practices from cultures around the world that have used herbs for generations to treat ailments like vertigo. Herbs such as ginger, ginkgo biloba, and peppermint are being studied for their potential to alleviate dizziness and improve circulation. This interest in time-tested remedies encourages a deeper exploration of how nature can provide solutions to modern health challenges.

In addition to herbal remedies, there is a growing emphasis on personalized wellness. Consumers are increasingly seeking tailored approaches to their health, recognizing that what works for one person may not necessarily work for another. This trend is particularly relevant in the context of vertigo, as various underlying factors can contribute to the condition. The use of personalized herbal supplements, guided by knowledgeable practitioners, can empower individuals to find the right combination of herbs that suit their unique needs and circumstances.

Mindfulness and lifestyle integration are also gaining prominence within the realm of natural healing. The recognition that mental and emotional well-being plays a crucial role in physical health has led to a more holistic view of treatment. Practices such as yoga, meditation, and breathwork are being incorporated alongside herbal remedies to create comprehensive strategies for managing vertigo. This multifaceted approach not only addresses the symptoms but also promotes overall wellness and resilience.

Lastly, the digital age has facilitated greater access to information and resources related to natural healing. Online platforms provide a wealth of knowledge about herbal remedies, user experiences, and research findings. This accessibility empowers individuals to make informed decisions about their health and encourages community engagement in sharing experiences and recommendations. As a result, the trend toward natural healing continues to flourish, offering hope and effective solutions for those seeking relief from vertigo.

Building a Community for Support

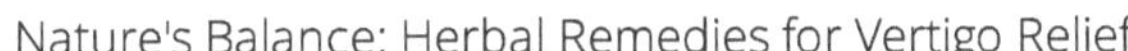

Nature's Balance: Herbal Remedies for Vertigo Relief

Building a community for support is essential for anyone navigating the challenges of vertigo. When individuals experience this condition, they often feel isolated and overwhelmed. Establishing a supportive network can provide not only emotional comfort but also practical advice and shared experiences that can enhance one's journey toward relief. By connecting with others who understand the nuances of vertigo, individuals can build relationships that foster healing and resilience.

An effective way to create this community is through local support groups or online forums focused on natural remedies and herbal supplements for vertigo relief. These platforms allow individuals to share their stories, discuss various treatments, and exchange tips on lifestyle adjustments that may alleviate symptoms. Engaging with others who are on similar paths can empower individuals to explore different herbal remedies, learn about new approaches, and gain insights into what has worked for others. This collective knowledge can be invaluable in finding effective solutions.

Additionally, workshops and educational events can be instrumental in building a community. Hosting or attending gatherings that focus on herbal remedies and holistic health can introduce individuals to new techniques and practices that support vertigo relief. Such events also create opportunities to meet practitioners and experts in the field, providing access to resources and information that may not be readily available otherwise. The sense of camaraderie that arises from these shared experiences can foster motivation and encouragement among participants.

Social media platforms can also play a significant role in cultivating a supportive community. By joining groups dedicated to natural health and wellness, individuals can access a wealth of information and connect with others who share their interests. These online communities often serve as safe spaces for discussions about personal journeys, challenges faced, and successes achieved, creating an environment where individuals can feel understood and valued. Sharing experiences in this manner can lead to the discovery of effective herbal supplements and remedies that may have been overlooked in traditional settings.

Ultimately, building a community for support not only enhances individual experiences with vertigo but also encourages a collective exploration of natural remedies. By uniting with others, individuals can share knowledge, inspire one another, and foster a sense of belonging. This community-driven approach not only helps individuals cope with their symptoms but also promotes a holistic understanding of health and wellness that is rooted in nature. Through collaboration and shared experiences, individuals can find strength and resilience in their journey toward relief from vertigo.

Chapter 10: Conclusion and Final Thoughts

Summary of Key Points

In "Nature's Balance: Herbal Remedies for Vertigo Relief," key insights emerge that underscore the importance of understanding the underlying causes of vertigo. This condition, often characterized by dizziness and a sense of spinning, can stem from various factors, including inner ear issues, migraines, or even anxiety. Recognizing these triggers is essential for anyone seeking effective natural remedies. By identifying the root cause, individuals can tailor their approach to treatment, making it more effective and personal.

The book emphasizes the role of herbal supplements in managing vertigo symptoms. Several herbs, such as ginger, ginkgo biloba, and peppermint, have been highlighted for their potential benefits. Ginger, for instance, is known for its anti-nausea properties, which can be particularly helpful during vertigo episodes. Ginkgo biloba is often praised for its ability to enhance blood circulation, potentially alleviating dizziness. By integrating these herbal remedies into daily routines, readers can explore a holistic approach to alleviating their symptoms.

Another vital point discussed is the importance of lifestyle modifications alongside herbal treatments. Simple changes, such as staying hydrated, practicing balance exercises, and managing stress through mindfulness techniques, can complement herbal remedies and enhance their effectiveness. The synergy between lifestyle adjustments and herbal supplements creates a comprehensive strategy for managing vertigo. This holistic approach not only addresses the symptoms but also promotes overall well-being. Education and awareness are crucial themes in the book. Understanding how various herbs interact with the body empowers individuals to make informed choices about their health. The text provides valuable information on dosage, preparation methods, and potential side effects of various herbal remedies. This knowledge equips readers to navigate their options confidently, ensuring that they can use herbal supplements safely and effectively.

In summary, "Nature's Balance" offers a wealth of information on natural remedies for vertigo relief. By recognizing the causes of vertigo, utilizing specific herbal supplements, making lifestyle adjustments, and educating themselves about these treatments, readers are empowered to take charge of their health. This multifaceted approach not only addresses the immediate symptoms of vertigo but also fosters a deeper understanding of one's body and health, paving the way for a balanced and harmonious life.

Encouragement for Self-Care

Self-care is an essential aspect of managing vertigo and promoting overall well-being. Taking the time to nurture oneself can significantly enhance the effectiveness of herbal remedies and natural treatments. By cultivating a routine that prioritizes both physical and mental health, individuals can create a supportive environment that fosters healing and balance. Remember, self-care is not merely a luxury; it is a necessity for those seeking relief from the challenges posed by vertigo.

Incorporating mindfulness practices into your daily routine can greatly improve your self-care efforts. Techniques such as meditation, deep breathing exercises, and gentle yoga can help ground you, reducing anxiety and promoting a sense of calm. These practices allow you to connect with your body and become more aware of your physical sensations, which can be particularly beneficial when dealing with the disorienting effects of vertigo. By focusing on your breath and being present in the moment, you can build resilience against the stress that often accompanies this condition.

Nutrition plays a crucial role in self-care, especially for those seeking natural remedies for vertigo. A balanced diet rich in whole foods, including fruits, vegetables, whole grains, and healthy fats, can provide the nutrients necessary for optimal brain and nerve function. Herbal supplements such as ginger, ginkgo biloba, and peppermint can also be incorporated into your diet to enhance circulation and reduce symptoms of vertigo. By being mindful of what you consume, you empower yourself to take control of your health and well-being.

Engaging in regular physical activity is another vital component of effective self-care. Gentle exercises, such as walking or swimming, can improve circulation and alleviate feelings of dizziness. Additionally, balance exercises can help strengthen the body's ability to manage spatial orientation. It is essential to listen to your body and find activities that feel right for you, incorporating movement that is both enjoyable and accessible. This not only promotes physical health but also uplifts your mood and fosters a sense of accomplishment.

Lastly, connecting with others can provide emotional support and enhance your self-care journey. Whether through support groups, friends, or family, sharing your experiences can help alleviate feelings of isolation and create a network of encouragement. Surrounding yourself with understanding individuals can be incredibly empowering, reminding you that you are not alone in your quest for relief from vertigo. Embrace the power of community as you navigate your path towards wellness, using both herbal remedies and self-care practices to restore balance in your life.

Resources for Further Learning

When exploring the world of herbal remedies for vertigo relief, it is beneficial to seek out a variety of resources that can deepen your understanding and enhance your experience. Books dedicated to herbal medicine and natural remedies can serve as invaluable guides. Titles such as "The Complete Herbal Handbook for Farm and Stable" by Juliette de Bairacli Levy or "Herbal Antibiotics" by Stephen Harrod Buhner provide insights into the benefits and applications of various herbs, including those specifically targeting vertigo. These texts offer foundational knowledge that can empower you to make informed decisions about your health.

Online platforms have become a treasure trove of information for those interested in natural remedies. Websites such as the American Herbalists Guild and the National Center for Complementary and Integrative Health provide research-based insights and articles on herbs and their effects. These resources often include case studies and personal testimonials that can lend additional credibility to the information presented. Engaging with online forums and communities dedicated to herbalism can also facilitate discussions and exchanges of experiences with others who share your interest in natural healing.

Courses and workshops focused on herbal medicine can offer hands-on experience and deeper learning opportunities. Many herbalists and wellness centers provide classes that cover the identification and preparation of herbs, as well as their medicinal properties. Participating in these educational experiences not only enhances your knowledge but also connects you with like-minded individuals and experts in the field. These interactions can lead to invaluable mentorship opportunities and provide a supportive network as you navigate your journey toward vertigo relief.

Podcasts and video channels focused on herbal remedies are another excellent way to absorb information in a more dynamic format. Numerous professionals in the field share their expertise through interviews, discussions, and practical demonstrations. This multimedia approach can cater to different learning styles, making it easier to grasp complex concepts related to herbal treatments. By following reputable sources, you can stay updated on the latest research and trends, ensuring that your knowledge remains current and relevant.

Lastly, local herbal shops and apothecaries often serve as both resources and community hubs. Engaging with knowledgeable staff can provide personalized advice tailored to your specific needs. Many shops also offer workshops or events that allow you to learn more about herbal remedies in a practical setting. By immersing yourself in these local resources, you can enhance your understanding of herbal supplements for vertigo relief while supporting your community and fostering connections with those who share your passion for natural healing.

Nature's Balance: Herbal Remedies for Vertigo Relief

Back Page Title

Lorem Ipsum is simply dummy text of the printing and typesetting industry. Lorem Ipsum has been the industry's standard dummy text ever since the 1500s, when an unknown printer took a galley of type and scrambled it to make a type specimen book. It has survived not only five centuries, but also the leap into electronic typesetting, remaining essentially unchanged. It was popularised in the 1960s with the release of Letraset sheets containing Lorem Ipsum passages, and more recently with desktop publishing software like Aldus PageMaker including versions of Lorem Ipsum.